CO-AVN-931

Delusion and Belief

LONDON : HUMPHREY MILFORD
OXFORD UNIVERSITY PRESS

Delusion and Belief

By

CHARLES MACFIE CAMPBELL

Professor of Psychiatry in Harvard Medical School
Harvard University

CAMBRIDGE

HARVARD UNIVERSITY PRESS

1927

PRINTED AT THE HARVARD UNIVERSITY PRESS
CAMBRIDGE, MASS., U.S.A.

Contents

Delusion and Belief

I

On the Biological Study
of Belief

MAN has long ceased to be the sport of inanimate nature; he has penetrated the laws of the physical world and harnessed its forces to his own designs. He is no longer impotent in face of the devastating forces of disease, but by mastering the nature of these forces and studying his own bodily resources, he has erected cunning defences. Encouraged by these triumphs, impatient at being himself the plaything of blind impulses, man feels renewed ambition to understand and control the forces which make up his own personality and determine his destiny.

The analysis of these forces and of their transformations brings one face to face with the varied beliefs of man and shows how much these beliefs contribute to the success or failure of the individual and of the group. Thus the study of beliefs is no academic discipline, but is part of the general study of the mechanisms of man's adaptation to his environment, conceived in the widest sense of the term.

In the biological study of the functions of an organism, it is useful by experimental procedure to isolate or to modify each function to be studied. In the study of belief this method is rarely available; even to acquire valuable knowledge it is not allowed to tamper experimentally with our fellows in regard to the main issues of human life. Biological study, however, learns much not only from the experiments of man but also from the experiments made by nature in the production of disease; the symptoms of disease have thrown much light on the dark places of human physiology.

Nature does not hesitate to tamper in the most drastic way with any of life's issues, or shrink from exposing human nature to the most searching tests. The careful analysis of these experiments made by nature, the scrutiny of various temperaments exposed to different moulding influences and critical experiences, and the study of the corresponding variations in belief, throw much light on the adaptive rôle of belief in general. In the light of such studies, familiar beliefs, hitherto taken for granted and exciting little curiosity, become fascinating examples of man's adaptation to his environment; they lose their static and absolute quality, and under the solvent of analysis may again become living and plastic, more efficient instruments for the purposes of the individual life.

4

II

Belief as an Important Topic of Hygiene

IN the past, students of health and students of belief have followed paths strangely remote from
each other; these paths now seem about to issue on
the broad highway followed by all students interested in human nature and its complicated problems. The term health begins to be more adequately conceived, and is seen to include sanity of
beliefs, as well as soundness of body; this is a return
to the earlier outlook, when the word *sanus* had the
same broad meaning, familiar to us in the phrase
mens sana in corpore sano. The divorce of the mental from the physical has been the source of grievous
errors; it would be well if, in discussing health, we
should think rather in terms of the complex ("mental") and the simple ("physical") functions of the
individual man.

Man not only strives to maintain his individual
existence and to propagate his kind, but he also
strives to attain happiness. He has to acquire and
assimilate food, to defend himself against noxious

organisms; and failure to perform these functions is paid for with his life; but the environment of man, to which he has to react, is not merely a source of supplies and the habitat of hostile organisms — it is a social environment permeated with spiritual forces which can never be expressed in simple material terms. The mechanisms by which he adapts himself to the simpler factors in the environment have been made the object of intensive study, and medicine can claim that it has increased the number of infants who survive, and has prolonged the span of the individual life. So far medicine has given scant consideration to the mechanisms by which man adapts himself to the social environment, and has tended to neglect the beliefs which play so large a rôle in this adaptation, objects of study as important as the simpler mechanisms by which he maintains his soundness of body.

If it be through the simpler mechanisms that he adds to the span of life, it is through the more complex mechanisms that he adds to its quality and gives to life its specific value. These beliefs, which give life its value, and do so much to determine the happiness of the individual and of the group, may also have much to do with the prolongation of life; the millions of men wiped out in the World War were not destroyed by famine or by pestilence, but because of the inadequacy of the complex mechan-

isms which determine man's beliefs and his behavior. Man's beliefs are thus seen to be not only a
question of happiness or unhappiness — they may
involve the issue of life or death, for the individual
and for the group. It is no mere theoretical task to
scrutinize man's beliefs and the factors which determine them; it has intensely practical bearings, it is
the most important and the most difficult task in
the field of public health. The medical profession
now boasts proudly of the quantitative addition it
has made to human life; the time may come when it
will point with equal pride to measures which have
added to the quality of human life, and which have
helped the individual and the group to deal more
sanely and soundly with those vital issues upon the
management of which the special significance and
value of human life depend. In these pages a few
such issues are discussed, with the help of some illus-
trative cases.

III

On the Relation of Delusion and Belief

THE concrete material referred to in the following pages has been chosen to illustrate the rôle of beliefs in the adaptation of the individual to the stresses of existence, and may serve to show that the delusions of the ill-balanced and the beliefs of the orthodox are more closely akin than is usually recognized. Under special strain the orthodox may lapse from conventional belief into individual delusion, and the delusion of one person, rejected by his contemporaries, may in another group or period become a socially acceptable belief. Delusion is no strange and mysterious element, it is no foreign parasite battening on the mind, it is not the meaningless expression of disturbed physiological processes; delusion is an attempt of the personality to deal with special difficulties, in which attempt the mind not infrequently tends to revert to primitive modes of adaptation, which are at variance with the actual level of thought of the period and group in which the individual finds himself; it is an attempt which has gone wrong in so far as it estranges the individual from his social group. Delusion, like fever, is to be looked on as part of nature's attempt at cure, an endeavor to neutralize some disturbing factor, to compensate for some handicap, to reconstruct a working contact with the group, which will still satisfy special needs. To those with no such special needs the delusion is apt to appear superfluous, repellent, grotesque; fantastic delusions are apt to excite laughter, although they may be the spontaneous attempts at self-cure of the bereaved, the childless, the thwarted, and the sensitive. By the medical profession the odd beliefs of the individual patient are not infrequently disposed of in a summary way as delusions, instead of being closely studied in relation to the underlying needs, for which perhaps much might be or might have been done. The lay attitude toward the more severe mental disorders, in which delusions play so large a rôle, is largely determined by this lack of insight into the deep human conflicts revealed by these very delusions. This lack of insight does much to maintain the artificial chasm which separates the mentally disordered from the sane. It does a grievous injustice to those suffering from mental disorders, and it prevents the ordinary man from seeing his own beliefs and those of other groups and other periods in correct relationship to the important forces which mould his life and the history of his group. With a fuller appreciation of the process by which the mentally disordered struggle, though unavailingly, to build up a universe which does justice to their needs, the more fortunate individual, whose beliefs are harmonious with those of his group, would be more likely to deal with problems of belief in general and with important social movements in an enlightened and constructive way.

IV

Some Important Issues in Life and Individual Modes of Dealing with them

Bereavement and Modes of Dealing with it

THERE is one test to which all are subjected — the test of bereavement. In face of the death of the beloved, no modification of the situation is possible. The human mind, however, does not remain completely passive in face of the blow, does not merely register it objectively and add this new datum to the accumulation of individual experience. The situation is not dealt with in a cold intellectual way, but is dealt with in the light of the emotional needs of the individual. Where there is some uncertainty about the death, in cases of shipwreck, etc., the friend most deeply attached to the dead person refuses to consider the death as a fact long after it has been accepted as such by those with less close emotional relationship. Even where the death is accepted as a fact, one hesitates to take the fact in its absolute implication, and this modification of the fact by thought is indicated by the language we use. We prefer to say, "he has passed away," instead of "he is dead." Complete annihilation of the individual we love may be intolerable to us; there persists the longing expressed by the poet,

> But oh for the touch of a vanished hand
> And the sound of a voice that is still.

Tennyson on the Death of his Friend Hallam

It is interesting to study the way in which different individuals at different periods and in different countries react to the situation. The poet utilizes the emotional intensity of the experience for a creative purpose, and weaves it into "In Memoriam," in which his thought wanders over a wide range and the immediate personal loss is seen in the perspective of man's destiny in general. He finds the current beliefs of his time an adequate resource in his time of trial, and by showing in appealing form their dynamic rôle, he makes a helpful contribution to the group; he makes the dead formulæ into a living truth.

Carlyle on the Death of his Wife

Carlyle, obsessed with regret and remorse, to a large extent limits himself in a characteristic way to the simple repetition of his expressions of grief: "Am of a sadness, and occasionally of a tenderness which surprises even myself in these late weeks . . . seems as if the spirit of my loved one were, in a poor metaphorical sense, always near me." [1]

One notes the reference to the nearness of the spirit of the loved one, corresponding to the strong emotional yearning; but either a lack of imagination or a rugged intellectual honesty makes the nearness of the spirit a merely metaphorical expression, to be strictly separated from the hard facts of experience.

Queen Victoria on the Death of the Prince Consort

Queen Victoria, the whole direction of her life upset by the death of the Prince Consort, carries on her work as if his spirit were near her, advising and directing her. It is possible that she would have admitted with Carlyle that the nearness of the spirit was merely a metaphorical expression for the longings of her own nature and the persistence in her mind of vivid memories. It is interesting to note, however, that something in her gave more than a mere metaphorical value to this expression: "The

[1] J. A. Froude, *Thomas Carlyle, A History of his Life in London, 1834–1881* (New York, Charles Scribner's Sons, 1910), ii, 303.

suite of rooms which Albert had occupied in the Castle was kept forever shut away from the eyes of any save the most privileged. Within these precincts everything remained as it had been at the Prince's death; but the mysterious preoccupation of Victoria had commanded that her husband's clothing should be laid afresh, each evening, upon the bed, and that, each evening, the water should be set ready in the basin, as if he were still alive; and this incredible rite was performed with scrupulous regularity for nearly forty years." [1]

How far can one deduce the belief of Queen Victoria from such behavior? Shall we take the behavior as expressive of her belief, or the formulation which she might have given, if she had been challenged on the topic? Perhaps in such a case we get a glimpse in the same individual of various levels of belief, and see that the more recent and more complex beliefs do not eliminate the more primitive types, but merely supersede them; under the stress of circumstances, the modern beliefs may not prove altogether adequate to the strain put upon human nature, which is glad to fall back upon more primitive formulations and behavior which, through countless generations, have served the needs of man.

[1] Lytton Strachey, *Queen Victoria*. New York, Harcourt, Brace and Company, 1921.

Hallucinatory Experiences after Bereavement

A similar situation is illustrated in the case of a woman in the prime of life suddenly bereft of her mother. After her mother's death she would go every evening to her mother's room and sit in her chair. She would have to sit in the room for at least ten minutes before she would hear her mother's voice; and then, as her mother would talk, she seemed to see her lying in bed just as she was before her death. The daughter would go to her mother's door every night to bid her good-night, and would frequently go into the room and sleep for some time and feel comfort and relief from these visits to the room which still seemed inhabited by the spirit of her mother.

It is worth noting that, while this woman had, in adult life, followed the orthodox religious beliefs of her community, she had as a child been taken by her mother to spiritualist meetings, and the grandmother, too, had been steeped in the same views. The patient, as a matter of fact, believed that spirits do return.

Another patient, suffering from a condition of depression, told an interesting episode which had occurred many years before. Her husband disliked the use of the term "good-bye" and said that he would only use it when taking a last farewell. One day news was brought to her that her husband had been suddenly killed. He had left her that morning after his usual salutation of temporary parting. The thought that he had left her for good without having said good-bye preoccupied her greatly, and her mind was not completely at rest. One night, as she lay in bed with her arms under the sheet, she felt a hand above the sheet take hold of hers and a voice seemed to say three times "Good-bye." She had the feeling that this was a final parting, and henceforth her mind was at rest.

Different Interpretations of Such Experiences

To some, such an experience appears to have the same objective value as the ordinary experiences of everyday life, and is used as evidence of some orderly frame of events behind that of our matter-of-fact world, but which seems to duplicate, in a shadowy way, the ordinary interests and behavior of suffering humanity. Unfamiliar with the laws of human thought in health and disease, to them such experiences seem quite out of keeping with the known laws of the work-a-day world. To others, such an experience seems quite in keeping with what we know of human nature, of the emotional life, of the creative imagination. Some familiarity with the analysis of human nature in its everyday struggles makes superfluous for the explanation of these phenomena the introduction of a secondary world or other world which duplicates the present world. The interpretation of such an experience in terms of some other world is due to two factors, first, the intensity of the emotional craving, and second lack of knowledge with regard to the laws of the human mind in the world of our ordinary experience. Where the emotional need and the underlying craving are intense, although perhaps not very manifest on the surface, they may dominate the interpretation even in face of considerable knowledge of the laws of the human mind. Where ignorance of the laws of the human mind is extreme then, even with little emotional craving but simply with mild surprise or fear at unusual happenings, one meets a naïve interpretation of the facts. In order that experiences such as those described above may be sensibly dealt with by the individual, and not become a stumbling block to others, two things are necessary: first, the dissemination of knowledge with regard to the laws of the human mind in health and disease, a problem of general education, and secondly, the recognition by the individual of the rôle which his emotional needs play in relation to his beliefs.

A Bereaved Japanese Mother and Primitive Religious Beliefs

O-Toyo,[1] a Japanese mother, within a period of three days was bereft of her husband and of her three-year-old child.

"One day she thought of a weird consolation, the evocation of the dead. . . . (To have the dead called back one must go to some priest — Buddhist or Shinto—who knows the rite of incantation. . . . The priest calls upon the name of the dead, and as he cries, the tone of his voice gradually changes until it becomes the very voice of the dead person, — for the ghost enters into him.) The priest, in a voice which she thought to be that of her little child, gave her comfort and told her: 'It is not kindness to mourn for the dead. Over the Rivers of Tears their silent road is; and when others weep, the flood of that river rises, and the soul cannot pass, but must wander to and fro.' From that hour she was not seen to weep."

From her belief and these rites, O-Toyo gained some consolation, but the narrator of the story adds: "Today these rites are not allowed by law. They once consoled; but the law is a good law, and

[1] Lafcadio Hearn, "The Nun of the Temple of Amida," in *Kokoro, Hints and Echoes of Japanese Inner Life*. Boston and New York, Houghton Mifflin Company, 1896.

just, — since there exist men willing to mock the divine which is in human hearts."

The fact that the law has forbidden these rites suggests that even to those of her own race and tradition it appeared that there might be a better way of consolation and one less liable to be abused through the frailty of the human intermediary. At least, in such a case as hers there was the guaranty of a priestly tradition and a professional relationship. In other places, consolation of a similar type has been offered by those with no such priestly office and no professional tradition, but endowed with a certain form of nervous instability, which favors the development of dissociated and automatic activities which strike those unacquainted with the laws of abnormal psychology as being of mysterious origin, just as in some places the epileptic fit is looked upon as the manifestation of divine forces.

A Bereaved European Mother and Crude Spiritualistic Beliefs

In a narrative of contemporary life in another environment,[1] we find Hélène Smith, a handsome medium of thirty, an employee in a commercial establishment, consoling, during a mediumistic séance, a widow who had three years earlier lost her

[1] Th. Flournoy, *Des Indes à la Planète Mars:* Étude sur un cas de somnambulisme avec glossolalie. Paris, Fischbacher.

only son, Alexis. The medium appears to be in a trance, is speaking an unknown jargon, which is considered by those present to be the language of the inhabitants of the planet Mars. As soon as the bereaved mother is placed beside the medium "immediately begins the most moving scene of reincarnation that one can imagine; Madame Mirbel is on her knees, sobbing violently, at the side of the son who is found again, who showers on her signs of the most profound affection, and caresses her hands exactly as he was wont to do during his last illness, while he speaks in the Martian language (*"tin is toutch"*) which the poor mother cannot understand, but to which an accent of extreme sweetness and touching intonation give the evident meaning of words of consolation and of filial tenderness."

The reaction of the reader to such a narrative will depend on many factors. The gentleman who made the observation found it "a moving scene of reincarnation." Others may rather be moved by a feeling of indignation. To many the ludicrous element stands out, although the grief of the bereaved mother prevents that from being a dominant reaction. Others may see in this little incident, where no commercial interest enters, something in itself not dangerous, but capable of becoming seriously detrimental in unscrupulous hands.

The Atmosphere of the Séance

Side by side with the above extract one may place the experience of an army officer.[1]

Lieutenant E. H. Jones, prisoner of war at Yozgad, in association with Lieutenant C. W. Hill, a sleight-of-hand expert, spent many months in bamboozling his fellow officers and Turkish jailers by means of the ouija board. They showed that "in the face of the most elaborate and persistent efforts to detect fraud it is possible to convert intelligent, scientific and otherwise highly educated men to spiritualism, by means of the arts and methods employed by 'mediums' in general." It is particularly illuminating that when, eighteen months later, Lieutenant Jones explained to one of his converts the details of his fraudulent procedure, the convert with a pitying smile rejected this confession, and maintained that a certain happy guess of the intelligent lieutenant was due to "unconscious telepathy."

The talented lieutenants had respect for the tragedies of human life. "In building up the reputation of our spooks there was one type of séance we did not encourage. We threw aside the strongest

[1] E. H. Jones Lt. I. A. R. O., *The Road to En-Dor, being an account of how two prisoners of war at Yozgad in Turkey won their way to freedom.* With illustrations by C. W. Hill Lt. R. A. F. London, John Lane, 1920.

weapon in the medium's armour. The emotional fog which blinds the critical faculty of the sitter is most valuable to the medium and it is quite easy to create. A 'Darling Boy' from a dead Mother, or a 'My Son' from a dead Father does it. But there were limits to which we could not go . . . nobody's dear dead was allowed to appear on the scene." After his prolonged experience of these matters from a very unusual angle, Lieutenant Jones concludes: "When in the atmosphere of the séance, men whose judgment one respects and whose mental powers one admires lose hold of the criteria of sane conclusions and construct for themselves a fantastic world on their new hypothesis. . . . If this book saves one widow from lightly trusting the exponents of a creed that is crass and vulgar and in truth nothing better than a confused materialism, or one bereaved mother from preferring the unwholesome excitement of the séance and the trivial babble of a hired trickster to the healing power of moral and religious reflection on the truths that give to human life its stability and worth — then the miseries and suffering through which we passed in our struggle for freedom will indeed have had a most ample reward."

Disturbing Effect of Spiritualistic Environment

One man's meat is another man's poison, and what one person can stand may be fatal to another. Easy access to alcoholic drinks may mean little to the robust members of a community, but may prove fatal to the personality of those less vigorously endowed. For the sake of the weaker members the more robust may even forego the pleasure that comes from this form of stimulation. So, with regard to the indulgence in certain forms of emotional stimulation, it is well to realize that some people can stand what others cannot.

A widow, worn out with nursing a daughter through a fatal illness, visits a sister who, with some friends, gets a certain thrill from toying with the ouija board. The latter invites the bereaved mother to experiment. In a few days the ouija board, under the fingers of the mother, who is in a condition of great emotional turmoil, begins to form messages from the departed husband, and in a few days she hears his voice continually, is living side by side with him, and is in full delirium, finally requiring to be nursed back to health in a hospital.

One wonders, therefore, whether to the widowed mother there is not available some surer source of consolation, some broader basis upon which she can reconstruct her life, some sounder outlook or belief, which will not only do justice to the memory of the beloved, but place it in the setting of a system which responds to all the demands of her nature. We have to realize that the needs of the individual are variable, that the possibility of a wide grasp and penetrating interpretation of experience is limited, that the environmental beliefs and systems which are available have their limitations and that it is not likely that individuals with different needs and different intellectual endowments and different situations will find one uniform system of beliefs adequate for all purposes. Beliefs are of necessity a function of the individual and of the trials to which his destiny exposes him.

V

Unsatisfied Love and Individual Modes of Dealing with it

THE examples given above may serve to show how human thought deals with the grim fact of bereavement. Through such beliefs as those discussed above, an otherwise intolerable situation becomes tolerable; with their aid the bereft one may carry on gallantly, while without them the everyday task would be impossible of accomplishment. The biological value of belief is at once apparent. It is true that in some of the cases mentioned the belief, useful though it appears to be, would be considered delusion by the impartial spectator. The important practical question arises whether, in the face of the needs of the individual, other beliefs might not have been available, of equal utility, but without the social drawback involved in the term delusion.

On Certain Psychological Disturbances, frequently Exploited

One factor in the séance at Geneva is of considerable interest. The medium was talking in an

unknown jargon, supposed to be the language of
the inhabitants of the planet Mars. In Geneva, in
1896, in this circle probably more interest was felt
in the planet Mars than in those factors which interested the early Christians. At Corinth, too, in
the early days of the Church, one was able to speak
in unknown tongues and was apparently proud of it,
although not claiming that it was the language of
the planet Mars. Paul admitted that he could
speak in this way more than all of them, as well he
might with his experience on the road to Damascus.
With his robust good sense, however, he tells the
Corinthians that God alone knows what they mean
when they are speaking in an unknown tongue, and
that, if one is going to be of use, he had better talk a
language intelligible to his fellowmen; "He that
speaketh in an unknown tongue edifies himself, but
he that prophesieth edifieth the Church." [1]

Again, in a different period and in another cli-
mate we meet similar manifestations. In New England, toward the end of the seventeenth century,
we find some rather unstable girls meeting with two
West Indian slaves in the house of Mr. Parris in
Salem.[2] The group practises palmistry, fortune-
telling, and various spiritualistic tricks. We hear of

[1] I Corinthians, xiv, 4.

[2] Charles W. Upham, *Salem Witchcraft*. Boston, Wiggin and
Lunt, 1867.

a variety of gestures and acrobatic postures. They utter meaningless sounds ("talk in unknown tongues"), undergo various contortions and spasms. These performances soon gained considerable prestige. The performers were now in the centre of the stage, and they responded to it. They began to shout with insolence in the Church; the girls had complete immunity, were supposed to be under a supernatural impulse. They were considered to be bewitched, and when asked who had bewitched them, they began to utter various names. This was the beginning of the persecution of various of those named, which terminated in the execution of nineteen persons.

The component factors of this historical incident are instructive — a small group of ill-balanced people, symptoms of nervous instability, misinterpretation by the medical and theological professions, underlying animosities with regard to land tenure and other personal matters, a severe and rigid system of religious beliefs.

The following case may illustrate the insufficiently known fact that phenomena which, in such a historical setting or in the more meretricious atmosphere of the mediumistic séance, may seriously disturb men's peace of mind, are frequently met with in the most matter-of-fact surroundings.

A woman in the forties, a Catholic who had been

divorced and remarried and therefore felt cut off from her Church, was unable to get along without some religious contact. Christian Science failed to make a deep appeal, New Thought had the same result, and finally the patient drifted into spiritualistic meetings. After some time she began to feel a twitching in the nerves of her head, which she attributed to the touch of the departed spirits. Automatic writing came with ease to her. If placed at a desk with a pencil in her hand, the hand would write messages which she attributed to external forces. At the same time she stated that she always had to have the ideas in her mind first before writing them, and that she thought she could control her automatic writing. The messages which the patient wrote were not of much importance, and she made no effort to exploit them, being more or less indifferent to the phenomenon. A more energetic and ambitious person, with greater cultural resources, and more emotional tension could have produced a much more dramatic picture.

One may pass to look at a few cases illustrating how human thought deals with difficulties in relation to some other fundamental problems.

A major force in human nature is that which attracts the individual toward the other sex, and leads toward mating. Under the influence of the organic promptings, the thought of the individual becomes occupied with this topic, and coöperates with the blind urge of passion in working out some practical form of realization. Obstacles, however, may stand in the way of this realization, obstacles inherent in the constitution of the individual or determined by an unkind fate, for not to all does Eros decree the happy accomplishment of love. In face of such obstacles in the real world human nature is not without resource, but by the alchemy of thought may transform the situation into one which makes life still worth living.

Beliefs Representing the Undisguised Fulfilment of Desire

Thus a young man of solitary disposition and of strict habits, shy and rather prudish, began to have experiences which for him had apparently complete objective value and did not seem to him to be the construction of repressed desires. He felt that he was more or less haunted. He became convinced that an unknown but very rich girl was after him: "her heart is talking to my heart." He heard her voice. He roamed through the house seeking this person. He felt that he was in special communication with heaven.

These experiences were not in dream or part of a delirious experience, but they were dovetailed into

the everyday world of ordinary experience of which
he still had a quite satisfactory grasp.

It is not only adolescents who in the face of a
stunted or starved emotional life resort to such beliefs. An unmarried woman of sixty-four began to
be disturbed by finding that she was the object of
attention of various men whom, as a matter of fact,
she did not see and whom she could not identify.
Voices, however, said they wanted her. She heard
the voices of the plotters arranging to take her away
in a yacht. Young millionaries in automobiles kept
circling round her place of residence. She was so
much afraid of being abducted and carried away in
the yacht that she appealed to the police for protection. The patient claimed that she had seen God,
the Virgin Mary, and the angels, and felt that this
was not insanity but was a gift given to her.

A shy young man in the thirties began to talk of
a flirtation which he had had with an actress. As a
matter of fact, he had not talked to her personally,
but he claimed that from the stage she had been
flirting with him. He was sure that she had fallen
in love with him. The fact that he had caused this
woman to fall in love with him showed him that he
was a self-ordained priest; "they call it a secret of
love." "Someone has said that whoever could make
a woman fall in love would be ruler of the earth."

In such a case we see how a shy and somewhat

unsuccessful man manages, by the magic of thought, to transform a rather dreary world into a place where he is an object of desire to women and where he has at the same time high religious value.

Notwithstanding his subjective interpretation of experience to meet his craving for love and prestige, this man has an otherwise clear grasp of the ordinary work-a-day world in which he lives.

A man in the forties was separated from his wife, partly on account of his belief in Christian Science. He felt that he had a special mission. He became convinced that he was married to a singer in the Christian Science Church. "It appeared to me that she reflected love back to me from her looks and glances while singing in the Church." He was convinced that he was "divinely united" to this woman in marriage. He had never talked to her, but he felt that there was a perfect understanding between them. He felt that he was telling her just what he was doing every day. He felt happy in the light that was reflected from her.

The same underlying forces, the same reaching out after satisfaction, the same blending of the fundamental instinctive craving with the more exalted religious aspirations, are seen in the case of an unmarried woman who claims that she has had several "spiritual lovers" who are priests, and that she is the wife of one of the priests. She has had nine children who are snakes. She claims that she is the Virgin Mary and God.

In such utterances we see the underlying forces formulated in expressions which in part recall the crude totem beliefs of primitive man rather than the formulations of a twentieth-century woman.

Another woman tells us of having, for three or four years, occasionally experienced a sort of electric shock announcing the coming of her lover. She read about psychology and magnetism and mysticism, and found that this peculiar experience was due to magnetism projected by will power. The patient told of having gone through a mental marriage service. For some time she had been in communication with her sweetheart by mental telepathy.

In regard to such phenomena as these the disturbing influence of strong emotion on objective logical thought is evident, and creative imagination driven by primitive needs dominates the scene. As to whether the resultant beliefs, the individual solution of the internal difficulties, will be acceptable to the group, that may depend upon the current views of the group, their level of culture, their personal participation in similar experiences. Thus, with regard to religious experiences, some will accept and some will reject their validity.

Episode of Nervous Instability with Religious Interpretation

In the midst of a period of religious turmoil (1818), Joseph Smith in his fifteenth year had a remarkable experience: "I was seized upon by some power which entirely overcame me, and had such an astonishing influence over me as to bind my tongue so that I could not speak. Thick darkness gathered round me, and it seemed to me for a time as if I were doomed to sudden destruction . . . just at this moment of great alarm, I saw a pillar of light exactly over my head, above the brightness of the sun, it descended gradually until it fell upon me. . . . I saw two personages, whose brightness and glory defied all description, standing above me in the air."

A Methodist preacher treated this communication with great contempt, saying that there are no such things as visions or revelations in these days; but this same experience was later accepted by others as being of extraordinary significance.

VI

The Longing of the Childless and Individual Modes of Dealing with it

AS in regard to the sexual demands, so in regard to the craving for children, one sees the emotional needs moulding belief, dominating the situation, sometimes interfering seriously with social adaptations, sometimes making it impossible. The mother, bereft of her children, may go to the spiritualistic séance and get comfort from an atmosphere that gives more body to her phantasies than is possible away from this special stage-setting and official encouragement. O-Toyo talks to the playthings of her dead child, and so identifies herself with the latter that she becomes one with the group of children who play in the Temple of Amida.

The Wish-Fulfilling Beliefs of a Childless Woman

Other women have not been so fortunate as to have had children; and to some the unsatisfied longing for children at length becomes intolerable and nature demands her rights, forcing thought to cooperate with her demands. So a childless woman astonished her husband one day by saying that she was going to the doctor to demand her child, and said that she was sure that this doctor, many years ago, had taken away her baby. She claimed that she had recently seen her baby, now grown to boyhood. As she gave fuller rein to her imagination and became less critical, she claimed that she had had a series of children. Her other desires took advantage of the abdication of the critical faculty to assert themselves, and some years later she claimed that she herself was the daughter of the Queen of Russia, that she had been stolen, when a child one year old, by the anarchists and given to Jewish people to be brought up as a poor Jewish girl.

VII

The Desire for Power and Individual Modes of Dealing with it

Beliefs with Regard to the Importance of the Self

IN the case of this childless Jewish woman who believed that she had had ten children and was of royal lineage, we see in her beliefs the expression of that tendency to self-assertion, that desire for superiority, that craving for power, which is a very fundamental element of human nature. Beliefs that are the expression of such longings frequently arise in those who at an earlier period have had to face a situation of real inferiority, and who have smarted under this inferiority, whether social, financial, physical, or racial. An inferiority may be a spur to ambition and bring out all the latent power of the individual. The race is not always to the swift nor the battle to the strong. Demosthenes might have been a poorer orator if the original speech impediment recorded by tradition had not been such a challenge to him. The feeling of inferiority plays an important rôle in the life of many, and compensatory day-dreams are very frequent. When the balance of the mental functions is upset, it is striking how frequently there comes to the surface the claim by the patient to be God or Christ. The claim is made irrespective of sex. The belief may be a mere transitory expression in the course of a fleeting delirium; it may, on the other hand, be a much more stable belief, which persists while the patient goes on with much of the routine of everyday life, even accepting his own name and family connections and ordinary relations in life.

Dissociated Phenomena

In many, the same trend of belief does not reach this intensity or give rise to a formulation which is so much at variance with the beliefs of one's fellows. There are many individuals who feel that they are inspired and have a definite message, and their claim, although not accepted at face value, does not necessarily cause offence. Schopenhauer claimed that the truth of what he had written was absolutely established because it had practically been inspired by the Holy Ghost. Many people have had on occasion a special conviction and absolute certainty welling up from deep sources in their personality, and giving a special stamp to their interests and activities and beliefs, and these *sub-*

37

conscious forces are felt by the individual as *extra-personal* factors, and may be attributed to God or the devil or to disembodied spirits.

There are some in whom there is not so much an episodic manifestation of these forces as a placid and continuing belief of the divine within them; these people may be of the salt of the earth.

The creative artist, like the philosopher Schopenhauer, frequently feels that his activity is directed by subconscious factors over which the writer or artist has little conscious control. Barrie talks as if it were almost another person who writes his works. Thackeray claimed that his literary creations lived out their lives irrespective of his control. R. L. Stevenson felt that much of his productive work was done below the level of clear conscious direction.

It is well to realize how frequent are these phenomena in the lives of productive people, so that, when similar phenomena are observed in another setting, we shall be on our guard against their undue exploitation.

Beliefs Compensating for Feelings of Inferiority in Various Spheres

TWO PRETENTIOUS AUTHORS

To come back from this digression on dissociated phenomena to the mode in which a feeling of inferiority may influence the attitude, the behavior, the beliefs of the individual, we may present briefly an account of the history of two individuals with very definite handicaps.

A young man with complete self-confidence, unable to see any abnormality in his own mental condition, erroneously thought that his father had a mental disorder, and that those in his environment were immoral. He felt that he had ability and power to advise the community, and he published a pamphlet on health and other pamphlets on love. The pamphlet on health "guarantees cure in any non-epidemic disease and assures to you long life and health by easy method." In the other pamphlets he gives dogmatically his views about love, courtship, and marriage, and gives advice in a somewhat pretentious way to those who are about to marry. The self-satisfied and superior attitude of the individual, accusing those around him and posing as a leader, is in striking contrast with his actual personal limitations. From early years he had suffered from deafness; pulmonary tuberculosis and a mental upset had put an end to his college training. On restoration to physical health, he had carried on unskilled work or lived with his people. The strong desire for success which inspired him was not quenched by the actual situation. He felt that success must be his, and with no training or competence in regard to dietetics, he felt that his individual experience entitled him to lay down the law on the subject, and published his pamphlet which guaranteed long life and health. He attributed such importance to his views that he referred to them as likely to upset and revolutionize present medical science.

A similar attitude of self-satisfaction and of emphasis on his own capacity was that of another author whose book, however, had never reached the stage of going to press. This patient had written two books, one a prose work, "How the Matrimonial Agency Failed," the other a poem called "Basic Aims," both very crude and pretentious productions. In a third book he was dealing with war, good, morality, sex distinctions, religious basis (? bias). The patient, an excellent craftsman, had invented an ingenious mechanism with serious destructive possibilities. He claimed that "it may be used to carry on an effective warfare against society without danger to one's self."

This pretentious author had from boyhood been deaf, and received little formal education. The real restrictions of his life fostered a tendency to daydream of great accomplishments. Although to outsiders a solitary and shy individual, he was arrogant in the family, used big words, studied some medicine and phrenology, dreamed of being a great inventor. Having little success with women, he got comfort by looking down upon them as intellectually not his peers; but he later tried to establish himself on a better footing by taking dancing lessons. His dancing evidently lacked grace and he had to hire partners. He consoled himself with the fact that nobody could develop his steps logically and that he was the fastest dancer in existence. His mechanical skill showed itself in various ways, and it was a special temptation to him to see in his most recent invention not merely a toy, but a weapon capable of drastic social application, "the only morally effective instrument which a man can have and is very important in the struggle against greed and the exploitation of the masses."

VIII

Man's Beliefs about the Mechanism of Nature and the Order of the Cosmos

THE beliefs discussed so far have been concerned with topics of high emotional value; they have their root in the emotional reaction to death of beloved ones, failure to bear children, unsatisfied love, ungratified ambition. It seems to us natural that in dealing with such personal matters the desires of the individual should exert a powerful influence, and that the attitudes and beliefs of the individual should have a strongly subjective note. We are not surprised to find that, where the cravings are strong and the personality has special limitations, the individual elaborates and clings to beliefs which his neighbours reject as morbid.

In regard to topics such as the above, agreement between those individuals with crying needs and those with gratified desires seems hardly to be expected; where the needs vary so much, there will the beliefs also vary, for the beliefs in the cases we have studied seem to be an important factor in the adaptation of each man to his own special situation.

Personal Factors in Scientific Convictions

It would seem, however, that when we take up beliefs dealing with the structure of the world around us, we should get free from the disturbing influences of subjective factors and find uniform beliefs, except in so far as intellectual errors might creep into the product.

Modern man, emancipated from crude superstitions, is apt to assume that the world of his experience is something quite apart from his personality, and to think that in the discovery and acceptance of the laws that govern the phenomena of nature, animate and inanimate, the emotional needs of the individual play no part. But the world of each man's experience is inevitably interwoven with and penetrated by the forces that make up his inner life; and even in regard to the detailed structure and working of nature, the needs of the individual tend to assert themselves. It is in vain that man with his intellectual ambitions yearns to get outside the sphere of his own experience to some absolute beyond; it is difficult enough for him to study some minor element in the cosmos, without the disturbing influence of an undue subjectivity. Even with the same data available and with a certain uniformity of cultural influences, what a bewildering variety of beliefs! Darwin sees animate nature working according to certain laws; Carlyle [1] rejects these laws with contempt. A certain John Hampden,[2] "educated at Oxford University," believes that the earth is flat, and shows the honesty of his conviction by backing it to the extent of five hundred pounds; Alfred Russel Wallace believes that man's opinions are determined by observation and logical thought, and naïvely sets out to demonstrate to John Hampden that the earth is round, with the result that he is persecuted by the latter for almost two decades.

Carlyle's Reaction to Darwin's Theory of Evolution

It is worth while dwelling a little on Carlyle's impassioned rejection of a belief which had so much to support it, and the data of which he refused even to consider.[3] It is interesting to find the painstaking and conscientious historian of Frederick the Great thus rejecting a biological view based upon the

[1] J. A. Froude, *op. cit.*, ii, 329, 330.

[2] A. R. Wallace, *My Life; a Record of Events and Opinions*, (London, Chapman and Hall, 1905), ii, 365.

[3] Darwin's opinion of Carlyle is of some interest in this connection: "His mind seemed to me a very narrow one, even if all branches of science, which he despised, are excluded. . . . He thought it a ridiculous thing that anyone should care whether a

laborious collection of data during many years by a competent worker who had devoted constant thought to the topic discussed.

Ordinary intellectual processes do not throw light upon this rejection. The immediate topic seems to be one in regard to which an objective judgment might well be expected. There is no topic, however, in regard to which the emotion of the individual may not be keenly aroused; and what to Darwin seemed a mere biological truth, to Carlyle was a mortal challenge, threatening to rob him of that which he clung to with the greatest pertinacity, as alone making his life worth living. He was never tired of preaching the moral order of the universe, its spiritual nature. This belief, to him, was an immediate necessity. One may speculate as to the psychological basis for the intensity of this belief; one might wonder whether it was some compensation for the crude material which he felt insistently in his own nature, as the rare ethics of Schopenhauer seem to be the compensation for a nature that was essentially harsh and unsympathetic. Whatever the source of his intense spiritual convictions, for Carlyle they were so important

glacier moved a little quicker or a little slower, or moved at all. As far as I could judge, I never met a man with a mind so ill-adapted for scientific research." *The Life and Letters of Charles Darwin*, i, 78.

that no belief apparently contradictory could be even given a hearing.

The years have passed, and many have found it possible to accept the spiritual nature of the universe, and at the same time to admit that there has been, throughout history, a gradual unfolding of this spiritual nature. It has been found possible to accept the data of historical investigation and, admitting the processes of evolution, to see that what finally becomes explicit in the higher must already be implicit in the lower and dare not be eliminated from the equation at any stage of the process.

The Prophet and the Scientist; Doctrine of Values and Doctrine of Facts

Thomas Carlyle and Charles Darwin each dealt with experience in the light of his own special equipment. They formulated the results of their experience in very different ways; but after all there arises the question whether we dare reject the contribution of either of these men.

To the individual who is especially interested in spiritual matters the prophet seems to contribute much more than the scientist. The truth burns at white heat, and he makes others vibrate to music to which they might otherwise be insensitive; but if this influence be due only to the strong emotional note of the prophet wrestling with his own needs, then, as the fire dies out, the next generation finds only a small amount of true ore, and a heavy mass of slag which neither heats nor lights. On the other hand, he who has contributed to sound knowledge, who has made a little clearer the structure of the universe, a little less obscure the history of the past, he who has increased the control of the blind forces of nature, has made a contribution to the living fabric of truth which sooner or later will be woven into the ordinary tissue of the thought of man. Prophets will still be needed to guide and to illuminate, but they will accept with thankfulness as part of their heritage from the past some of the beliefs which their predecessors contemptuously rejected.

The Beliefs of Alfred Russel Wallace

Reference has already been made to Alfred Russel Wallace, the distinguished naturalist who, in 1858, independently, discovered the same important biological law as Darwin — the theory of natural selection. ("The Tendency of Varieties to depart indefinitely from the Original Type.") To Wallace the laws of evolution were altogether acceptable and conflicted with no doctrines with which he had emphatically identified himself. It is interesting to see how Wallace dealt with other problems of experience and with what intensity he clung to his views. He was treated for a chronic complaint by an American medium and believed that he derived great benefit. He was very much struck by the fact that this medium had given two evidences of "genuine clairvoyance" in predicting that (1) change of air would do good to his boy, and (2) within some time Wallace would see less of a lady friend. He believed that the cures at Lourdes are due to "one of the myriad forms of spirit agency." He was an inveterate enemy of vaccination. He wrote "Vaccination a Delusion: its Penal Enforcement a Crime, proved by the Official Evidence in the Reports of the Royal Commission." He felt that this was one of the most truly scientific of his works, adding somewhat pathetically, "the difficulty is to get it read." He was a vegetarian on principle, believing that "it will certainly be the diet of the future"; as a matter of fact, he throve better on a meat diet. He wrote an article to indicate how the Sabbath should be kept, and in it the reasoning was so unanswerable that "a well-known writer was so impressed by it that he made his own bed the following Sunday in accordance with its suggestions." Wallace attended many spiritualistic séances in England and in America. He narrates, in great detail, the various phenomena observed; tambourines playing, bells rung, messages written, waistcoats mysteriously removed. He was pro-

48

foundly impressed by figures at these séances issu-
ing from behind curtains — Indians, female figures
of various heights, even one carrying a real baby,
little girls, etc. When Wallace, confronted by one
of these figures, asked, "Is it Algernon?" the figure
nodded earnestly. This "recognition" (!) made a
deep impression on Wallace.

The case of Wallace illustrates the rôle played by
the individual personality in determining beliefs
even with regard to minor details of the mechanism
of the universe.

Even when beliefs on very limited topics may
have been more or less incidentally arrived at, they
are apt to be considered essential parts of our being,
not provisional coverings to be thrown aside later
for better-fitting garments; as the offspring of our
spirit, they are defended with tooth and nail.

If the personality enters so vigorously into beliefs
of such limited scope, beliefs dealing with the detailed mechanisms in nature, this is also true in regard to the beliefs or attitudes toward nature as a
whole, toward the cosmos of which we form a part;
it is true not only of those complex attitudes which
we call beliefs — it is true of the simpler experiences
to which we refer as perceptions.

Personal Factors in Simple Perceptions

We talk as if the perceptions (or percepts) of different people were the same, whereas there enters into each perception the whole individual with his complex personality, and two experiences denoted by the same word may be extremely divergent.

The skylark of Shelley is a blithe spirit; it is experienced by the poet in a different way from that in which it is experienced by the naturalist who identifies and classifies and perhaps stuffs it. The daffodils of Wordsworth, laughing and dancing in the breeze, are seen by him to form a jocund company, because the poet is in a gay mood and in his experience with the daffodils the gaiety is felt as part of the total experience, and it is as natural for him to see the gaiety in the daffodils as to see it in himself.

With a similar failure to distinguish between the subjective and objective, a young woman, torn between conflicting tendencies in her nature, talks of some vague conflict going on in the world at large, where antagonistic forces are at war. Another patient talks of guilt being in the air, while he feels that he himself is free from any suspicion of wrongdoing owing to the strictness of his life. One may call these reactions delusions, but they seem to represent the same mode of dealing with experience as that of the poet who finds the daffodils such charming company. Neither makes a strict distinction between subjective and objective. The poet, it is true, while responding to the environment under the inevitable restrictions of his own individual endowment, weaves his personal experience into poetical form, which gives it special charm, and which helps us to recreate the same experience in our imagination and to vibrate in sympathy with him. The poet makes of his individual experience something which can be utilized by others, which has social value, which does not estrange him from his fellows, which lasts so long as the mode of experience to which he appeals has not been stifled by purely utilitarian considerations. A poet laughing merrily in company with some daffodils by the roadside would, no doubt, be looked upon with great suspicion by the motorist, absorbed in the performance of his car or in calculations connected with industry or the stock exchange. Which of the two has the more adequate grasp of reality?

As with animate nature, so with inanimate nature, even modern man may feel a very marked kinship; or, rather, he may see penetrating what he beholds the same emotional forces of which he has himself immediate experience. The cloud of Shelley is not the cloud of the meteorologist, but it is something imbued with complex emotional values. To the adolescent lover the whole world is glowing with a romantic light and is full of tender meanings; to the devout believer with soul full of fervor the world is permeated with the spirit of the benign Deity, who is equally to be seen in the sunset glow and in the heart of man.

> Father and Friend, thy light, thy love
> Beaming through all thy works, we see,
> Thy glory gilds the heavens above,
> And all the earth is full of thee.

In regard to the skylark, the cloud, the daffodils, we seldom think of the dissimilarity of the experience of different individuals, which is covered up by the use of the same terms that are used for very different experiences, and by the fact that one can refer back from the verbal symbol used to the real object, which plays very much the same rôle in regard to the primary practical needs of all.

The extraordinary dissimilarity of the experiences of the lover, the poet, the divine, the stockbroker, face to face with the simple phenomena of nature, shows us that the human mind is no mere registering machine, no photographic camera; the simple perceptions, the complex beliefs of the individual are both impregnated with the total personality.

In the perceptions and beliefs of the most matter

of fact individual there seem to be episodic glimpses of that communion with Nature, that imperfect separation of the individual from the continuum in which he is bathed, which makes him unconsciously look upon the forces that permeate nature and those that permeate himself as identical and continuous, as if he himself were merely a small nodal point on the infinite meshwork of cosmic forces, a nodal point in which these forces somehow or other manifest themselves in that irreducible experience called consciousness.

Primitive Mentality, its Persistence in Modern Thought

This identification of himself with the forces around seems to represent a deep-seated level of modern thought, an ancient mode of experience, and can be correctly appreciated only if we consider in some detail the attitude of primitive man to the cosmic forces in the midst of which he finds himself involved as a constituent element.[1]

It is not possible for those who are accustomed to think in clearly defined concepts of a physico-chemical universe, organized according to certain causal relationships, to enter into the mind of primi-

[1] The general point of view here outlined is that of Lévy-Bruhl, as outlined in his *Primitive Mentality*, who is somewhat at variance with the English school of anthropologists.

tive man, for whom the concept of causality in our sense may have no meaning, for whom in general clearly defined concepts do not exist, whose method of thought is so much less differentiated than that of modern man, and who lives his experience rather than thinks it out in the discriminating mode of modern civilized man.

Primitive man has not come to emphasize, as does modern man, the contrast between the subject who thinks and the object he deals with; he has not withdrawn from the cosmos those forces of which he has immediate consciousness in himself; he has not withdrawn thought and feeling and will from the nature that surrounds him, and has not claimed them as his monopoly and correlated them with a highly organized brain. The energy of which he has immediate consciousness in himself has intimate connection with the energy which flows through all things. He is thus only imperfectly separated from surrounding nature. The sun, the stars, the rocks, the trees, the wind, the rain, the plants and animals all participate in his nature. Not only does their behavior have an immediate influence on him, but in virtue of his participation in the world process he can bend the cosmic forces this way and that, as electrical forces passing through a point may be there deflected throughout infinite space. So can primitive man by his behavior, by moulding the forces that permeate him, determine the occurrence of rain, the reproduction of animals, the fertility of the soil, the success of the hunt. Even twentieth-century man whistling becalmed for a breeze is unconsciously demonstrating this primitive attitude of mystical participation in the forces of nature.

Beneath the surface of our conscious life, with its logical canons and its insistence on causality, primitive man still lives out his communion with nature, still feels his kinship with sun and rain and totem animal, still feels that by bending the forces that pulse through him he can modify the manifestation of these forces in external nature. Caliban may seldom be allowed to roam above the surface, but when special stresses weaken his restraining bonds, he may again appear in the open. Then we find the man of culture indulging in statements that leave those around him perplexed, and in which they see neither rhyme nor reason. It is only when we remember the mode in which primitive man deals with experience, and realize the tendency of the primitive to lurk concealed beneath the surface of later modes of thought, that we get some insight into such beliefs as those of the following individual.

Mental Disorder Allowing Primitive Mentality to Express itself

An intelligent woman, who for some years had suspected hostility and criticism and crafty manœuvres around her, passed through an episode of acute mental disturbance, during which her view of the outside world was of very great interest. She felt a strange communion between herself and nature. The world outside had regained some of those wonders which it had for primitive man. The planets again had emotion. She had a certain responsibility for keeping the heavenly machinery going, just as primitive man is responsible, by his magic rites, for keeping alive the rhythm of the seasons, the reproduction of animals, the fall of the rain. She said, "I must keep the sun going." She felt that she could give life to the sun; by her looking at it, it seemed to increase in size. "I thought everything was animated, that the animals had a spirit that understood us. I felt a great kinship between the animal world and myself. I looked at the horses on the bridle-path and they seemed to prance — I thought matter was alive; I thought planets were jealous like human beings."

A wonderful example of the way in which the subjective mood of the individual colors the objective world of experience is seen in her statement, "If I marry just the right man everything will be all right, if not, the end of the world will be, the ice age, all cold." The principle is the same that is exemplified in the simple statement of Queen Victoria, heart-broken by the death of the Prince Consort, "The world is at an end for me." It seems unimportant whether the catastrophic experience is referred to as involving the structure of the cosmos or the soul of the individual; it is all one.

Participation in the Cosmic Process and Participation in the Ethical Process

As primitive man feels his mystic participation in the forces of the cosmic process, and bends them this way or that in view of the personal stake he has in the game, so civilized man, in whom the cosmic forces have developed self-consciousness, feels a participation in the ethical forces of the universe, and feels not only that they have an immediate influence on his own individual destiny, but that, in virtue of his personal stake, he is bound to bend them this way or that, that he somehow or other has a serious individual stake in the moral order of the universe, and is responsible for the way he deals with those forces that permeate his being.

Experience of Reality in Religious Ecstasy

Primitive man can hardly be said to believe, in the sense of giving a definite assent to a proposition with regard to objective relations; for him, experience with its relations brings its own conviction with it, and he enters into the experience drenched with certain emotional values and tendencies to reaction which are involved in the life of those around him, whose influence has moulded him since infancy. Perhaps the nearest approach to such an attitude is experienced by modern man in the condition of religious ecstasy, in which there is no strict separation between subject and object; in such a condition reality seems to be grasped in a special way, and the fullest conviction is attained, while formulation of it in clean-cut concepts and propositions is impossible. In the transport of love or the exaltation of the spiritualistic séance we see analogous phenomena. Thus, where deep emotions are stirred, the mode of reaction of the individual is liable to be nearer the attitude of primitive man, for whom the demands of logical thought have not yet become binding.

What is of importance to notice is that it is in just these states that we seem to be in closest contact with reality, and to grasp it more intimately

than in the condition of knowledge so important
for utilitarian purposes, where reality is objectified
and separated from the individual. Modern rational knowledge of God removes him further from
us than that more primitive experience, in which we
have immediate contact with him. The yearning
for a more intimate union with God than the intel-
lect can yield is very persistent; even beneath his
agnostic and detached attitude man still craves to
be at one with God, to return to that intimate communion with the cosmos which is more familiar to
the experience of primitive than to that of civilized
man.

IX

On the Mental Health of the Individual and of the Group

The Individual and Social Importance of Beliefs

HEALTH, mental and physical, is a topic of general interest, the discussion of which is an agreeable mental pastime; there are many, however, who look eagerly to such a discussion as that in the preceding pages for help in the practical direction of life. Even though handicapped by serious physical ailments, man may through his beliefs snatch success out of the jaws of defeat; and, on the other hand, man may be crippled through distorted beliefs, no matter what his endowment in strength and symmetry of body. The individual finds it good to be relieved from pain and other simple handicaps, but the measure of his life is the spirit that inspires it, and the scheme of values that directs its output of energy. In the community the worship of efficiency may lead to so-called progress, to the accumulation of material facilities and of serviceable knowledge, but these may be a blessing or a curse according as the beliefs which animate the community are sound or distorted; chemistry may be the handmaid of war as of peace, and wealth of material resources may either relieve or cumber the spirit. For the individual as for the community there is no more vital issue than his scheme of values, and to this the science of health has its contribution to make.

Health has a positive as well as a negative aspect; it means more than a freedom from recognized disease, — it means living out the endowment of the individual and of the group to the fullness of its capacity, — and the mental or spiritual functions are as much part of the endowment of man as the simpler or bodily functions. Merely to rub along is not healthy enough, if a higher level of attainment be within reach.

The social functions of the individual are as essential a part of his nature as the simpler self-preserving functions; they are perhaps best looked on as the fullest evolution of the latter. Any personal adaptation which seriously limits the social adaptation of the individual, which isolates him or estranges him or puts him in opposition to his fellows (not merely in opposition to his contemporaries, for in the course of time it may be found that he has really been in harmony with his fellows of a later age, while his contemporaries had not been conscious of their own potentialities), is to be looked on as an inferior level of adaptation, even although it may bring individual comfort or a transitory equilibrium; and the practical question arises whether a better level might not have been attained. The individual with a belief in eccentric dietetic fads, in fantastic schemes of perpetual motion, in naïve and primitive formulations with regard to the present structure of the earth (for example, John Hampden), the past history of life on this planet, the happenings after death, may thereby attain a certain degree of personal comfort, but as a social unit his usefulness may be restricted. Quite apart from the restriction of the life of the individual with such beliefs, these beliefs may become a focus of infection of considerable significance; they may give rise to waves of religious fanaticism, to social movements of anarchic or regressive tendency, to pernicious opposition to health movements (for example, anti-vaccination, Christian Science), to minor disturbing movements such as periodic waves of spiritualism, to major racial or national movements which lead to pogroms, lynchings, and wars of extermination.

The Diversity of Beliefs

The diversity of beliefs in relation to all issues of life is notorious; *quot homines, tot sententiæ*. The diversity depends upon such factors as general level of culture (savage, barbarian, civilized) and the accidents of historical development, upon race and environmental factors, and in the individual upon special temperament, special experiences, and special emotional needs. Experience teaches that no one system of beliefs can be looked upon as adapted to the infinitely varying needs of man at diverse levels of culture. Toleration of the beliefs of others, and recognition of the part which these beliefs play in the adaptation of others to their individual and group problems, are to be recommended. We are too apt to consider our personal beliefs, the beliefs of our caste, our race, our nation, as the only tenable and rational ones, which it is our duty to impose on others; orthodoxy is our system of beliefs, heterodoxy the views of others.

Toleration and Indifference not the Same

Toleration and indifference, however, are not the same; and while we may tolerate certain beliefs and see their rôle in the adaptation of the individual, we may also see the possibility of putting that adaptation on a different level; and the science of hygiene may look upon it as a most fundamental responsibility to do its best, so that the inferior adaptation of the individual who fails to utilize fully his possibilities may be raised to a different plane. This may be looked upon as the highest task of hygiene.

In the presence of O-Toyo robbed of her child we may consider the possibility of bringing to her consolation, which is not weakened by admixture with an unsound dramatic element and by primitive animistic conceptions. The frank expression of human sympathy has healing power; [1] a broader outlook on man's destiny can in some be cultivated; wise counsel may suggest productive activities giving a useful outlet to a mother's tender sentiments towards the young and dependent. Such help may enable her to bear her burden and may strengthen not weaken her fellowship with the group; it may develop certain latent possibilities within her, social reserves which so frequently atrophy when individual comfort is provided and when the self-seeking trends are able to monopolize successfully the energy of the individual.

[1] "Affliction's sons are brothers in distress
A brother to relieve, how exquisite the bliss."

The Optimum Belief Attainable by the Individual Varies with Several Factors

To give O-Toyo a broader and deeper grasp may, however, prove an idle dream. Primitive formulations may have too strong a hold on her; her whole mentality from childhood may have been so drenched in certain modes of dealing with experience that her beliefs cannot be transformed or developed; she is at one with her environment, and with its beliefs as embodied in language, folk-lore, tradition, and religion. Her mental endowment can assimilate only consolation presented in a naïve way. She may need the concrete, the vivid, the dramatic, to receive that comfort which may come to others from abstract and lofty formulations. It is wise to realize the limitations imposed on beliefs by racial traits, individual endowment, environmental culture. We see drawbacks in such restrictions of thought, but realize that even at the lower level comforting beliefs play a useful rôle. Unless we can furnish O-Toyo a more enduring consolation, which offers the possibility of carrying on her life without withdrawing from the fellowship of the group, it is of little use to emphasize the fact that her consolations are not those that we use. Her formulæ may not fit into our religious creed, or into our conception of cosmic relations; let us be glad that for O-Toyo there are resources available which make life still bearable. Let us leave her undisturbed in her beliefs, not tampering with instruments which to her are so valuable.

Inferior Beliefs due to Poor Habits of Thought

With the group typified by Mme. Mirbel of Geneva the situation is somewhat different. The belief in the reincarnation of her son, the indulgence in the stimulation of the spiritualistic drama, are in appearance of the same stuff as the experiences of O-Toyo; they seem to deserve the same toleration, and the same immunity from interference.

But Mme. Mirbel has had wider resources placed at her disposal; with different cultural opportunities, her mode of thought has not been so saturated in early life with the primitive conceptions of O-Toyo's environment. In face of her personal grief, more varied social outlets for her human affections are available; she has been supplied with a more generous store of information, a fuller training, more advanced cultural beliefs, a religion of broader outlook which does fuller justice to the mysteries of life and death. In the face of her bereavement, is all this equipment to be discarded, and is it necessary for her to fall back on the more primitive adaptation of O-Toyo? Is she not capable of a more mature and efficient adaptation? Or have we to recognize that she is as simple a soul as O-Toyo? We are apt to ignore the fact that while many a simple soul rides in a modern automobile, and listens with pleasure to the radio, talking the language of modern culture, utilizing its extraordinary material resources, her personal cultural level may correspond to that of O-Toyo. There are some to whom the cultural beliefs of their group are external garments rather than part of the fibre of their being; in face of a serious demand the formal garments are discarded, and they fall back on their more primitive resources.

Progress to be Attained by Spreading Information and Cultivating Better Habits of Thought

Those interested in the healthy development of the community cannot regard such a regression to primitive levels with indifference. In the individual case it may be tolerated as the best adaptation attainable by a rather defective endowment, but it can only be regretted in the case of those of better endowment. One does not wish to rob souls in trouble of their comforting beliefs, but one may strive to put at their disposal beliefs more in keeping with the culture of their period and environment than the formulæ of primitive man. The formulæ of their religion can perhaps be rendered more living to them, so that, even if they do not grasp religious truths in the same penetrating way as others, they may find in these truths at the same time a source of comfort and an instrument of social solidarity. In the case of many people with fair endowment, the lapse into the primitive, the lazy acceptance of the crude, can be traced to poor habits of thought, to continued indulgence in the habit of wishful thinking instead of the utilization of thought for facing facts and dealing with situations in a realistic and purposeful way. This latter mode of thought enables the individual to extend the horizon of his interests, to dive a little deeper into the stream of social life, to use spiritual beliefs not merely for conjuring up a pleasing cosmic picture, but as an incitement to a fuller participation in the ethical process of the universe.

This more mature and healthier mode of dealing with the situation can be encouraged not only by some attention in the formative period to the danger of wishful thinking, but also by the dissemination of sound information. Many would be safeguarded from perplexity over spiritualistic claims, if they knew more about the reactions of the nervously unstable. They know that epileptics are sick people, not specially qualified as priests to interpret the deepest mysteries. So if the wayward reactions of the hysterical, of the pathologically romantic and of the unscrupulous, were recognized as ordinary medical and psychological problems, the medium would, as a rule, come to be looked on with sympathy as a person not to be exploited, frequently a problem for the doctor, sometimes a problem for the police if deliberately exploiting others. She would cease to be looked on as the chosen vehicle of spiritual powers save by the ignorant and the incurably credulous. Whoever does anything wittingly or unwittingly to increase the prestige of such false prophets is doing a subtle disservice to the mental health of his community. With toleration for those who, through poor endowment, lack of information, or terrible bereavement, cling to such beliefs, it still behooves us to do what is possible to prevent others, capable of a better adaptation, from accepting as adequate these primitive formulations.

Inferior Beliefs about Health; their Danger to the Group

In a similar spirit of toleration, but not of acceptance or indifference, one may meet such problems as those presented by Christian Science [1] and other

---

[1] As many lowly animals survive by virtue of their mimicry or coloring, through which they avoid notice or are mistaken for quite different animals, so it has been suggested that Christian

peculiar health cults. People suffering from ailments and distress of various kinds have, with the help of such beliefs, managed to get personal comfort and to return to fuller social activity. Where the beliefs seem to be thus helpful and to represent progress from previous invalidism, it might seem injudicious to interfere; but the question is, whether the individual is living up to the full measure of his health, including the healthy use of his higher mental functions, so long as he leans upon such a series of beliefs. One would like to maintain the gain of escape from invalidism, while avoiding payment in the form of acceptance of an attitude or belief which represents an inferior utilization of the higher functions. Can it be looked on as a healthy utilization of the higher functions to be blind to the facts of disease, to ignore a vast body of information painfully accumulated, to discourage the putting of thoughtful questions to nature by way of experiment, to treat as non-existent the grim and continual struggle between man's complex organism and the destructive germs that are around him, between the healthy tissues of the body and the aberrant tissues that tend to become destructive

Science partly owes its survival to the protective mimicry involved in the name through which at the same time it simulates a religion and a science. Its claim to either of these titles it would be difficult to substantiate.

70

growths? The higher functions of thought find
their healthy expression when, in face of difficulty,
thwarting, bereavement, they are utilized to scrutinize carefully the facts of the situation, to see how
far they are open to modification, to elaborate with
all available resources appropriate means to meet
the difficulty. It cannot be looked on as healthy to
find personal comfort by seeing the world in the
light of our desire, and saying that something is not
when it is. Those who have found personal comfort
and increased efficiency through Christian Science
have found it largely by adopting the healthy attitude that, even when there is some physical ailment,
it is often better to ignore it and to go on playing
the game of life. The healthy emphasis on the main
issues of life enables many people to get along with
physical ailments to which others are devoting an
unhealthy amount of attention. Thus to ignore
certain physical ailments, after reasonable practical
steps have been taken, — to treat them with judi-
cious neglect, — is a different matter from saying
that they do not exist; and it is not necessary to en-
cumber a healthy attitude of emphasis on the
positive aspect of life with a pretentious pseudo-
religion.

For this community it would be a serious matter if
this facile blindness to disagreeable facts were to become widespread, and if, in face of the constant ag-

gressiveness of disease-bearing forces, the thoughtful and consistent study of health problems and of practical health measures were to be weakened. Protected by the efforts of their healthier-minded fellows, the Christian Scientists can bask in their illusions; but it is perhaps necessary to realize the latent danger which they represent, and to see that a spread of their point of view under the influence of some dominant personality might lead to serious consequences, to impairment of public health activity, to devastating epidemics. One would wish to raise the level of thought of such a group to a healthier level without the stimulus of a major epidemic. The optimist takes it for granted that man is progressively and automatically becoming more reasonable, and that with the spread of education all such problems will be automatically solved. On the other hand, it is disconcerting to see that such beliefs as those of Christian Science are not limited to the illiterate or poorly educated, but are found at all levels; wishful thinking is by no means rare even in academic circles.

Inferior Beliefs about Social Problems

The type of reaction shown by the Christian Science group in regard to the disagreeable facts of individual disease may be shown by others in regard to disagreeable facts of the community life. There are some who prefer not to see the facts of contemporary life, except in the light of their desire, with the vice gilded over, inequality and injustice nonexistent, the ornamental and comfortable in the foreground. Progress is taken for granted, dangerous regressive forces are smiled at; it is assumed that man has progressed in his scheme of values and in his personality as much as in his knowledge and control of material resources; even the World War has not dampened such optimism.

The danger of such wishful thinking in the social sphere, as in regard to disease, is that it may similarly discourage the healthy application of the realistic function of thought to the accurate observation of facts and to experimental study and investigation of the underlying laws. Through such studies man, in his group organization, may hope to grapple in an adequate way with the real facts of existence, with poverty, crime, inequality, injustice, political chicanery, class and racial antagonism. It needs all the resources of thought to deal with the infinitely complex social problems of a highly industrialized environment, of somewhat heterogeneous racial composition, in which the binding influence of the customs and traditions of more primitive communities has been dissolved while no serious substitutes have been established.

In regard to still wider relationships the same

principles are seen to apply; the optimist talks of universal peace, seeing the immediate future of this planet in the light of his desire, and often denies the existence of harsh realities, the different cultural levels of different races, antagonistic modes of thought, ingrained nationalisms, economic rivalries, traditional hates. To deal with such actualities all the resources of thought of the community are required, and much more expenditure of energy than is necessary to get immediate satisfaction by the indulgence of pleasing day-dreams.

Emphasis has been laid above on the tendency in the human mind to see the world in the light of our desire. This tendency may get the upper hand to an unhealthy degree; it may lead to wilful blindness and lazy optimism, while the facts demand sweat and blood. Even the insistence on the spiritual order of the universe may be associated with an attitude of complacent contemplation of the ideal reality behind the crude actualities of the work-a-day world, in which attitude the latter lose all importance and elicit no strenuous endeavor. Thus early Christianity recommended a complete withdrawal from participation in ordinary affairs, even from reproduction of one's kind — a recommendation rejected by human nature, impelled by other forces to fulfil its destiny.

Emphasis on the ideal world behind the confused

world of phenomena need not develop an attitude of indifference toward everyday experience, or paralyze man's efforts to mould the forces in which he finds himself involved. The spiritual order of the universe may be regarded, not as something detached and apart from the world of our experience, but as the latter world more adequately conceived; and it may be realized that only through the medium of this world can we participate in that ethical process of which we have an intuitive conviction.

The belief in the spiritual order of the universe is, from the point of view of the health of the individual and the group, an important driving force; it encourages the maximum output of energy, it supports social solidarity, it compensates for the recognition of one's own handicaps, it supports the individual during transitory discouragement, through thwarted hopes, and helps him to suffer the "slings and arrows of outrageous fortune," while at the same time urging him

> . . . to take arms against a sea of troubles
> And by opposing end them.

Beliefs such as the above have been a source of untold strength to individuals and nations. The prophets who have stimulated these beliefs, given them vitality and actuality, have been a source of strength to their community, supplying it with

75

spiritual vitamines. The general belief in a spiritual interpretation of the world will be precipitated in different forms in different periods and different climes; it may be expressed in the creed of a church, the philosophy of a thinker, the creation of a poet. It will be grasped in a more meagre sense or in its fuller bearing according to the cultural level, the personal endowment, the intellectual training of the individual; it will be colored by innumerable influences, will contain various inclusions and residuals. But as a health factor, as a dynamic component, the exact formulation is unimportant compared with the general belief or attitude. The intuitive conviction of man in relation to this matter, receiving ever clearer formulation as his evolution has progressed, is a datum of basic significance. It represents a tendency as fundamental in human nature as the tendency of life to perpetuate itself, and as little open to further analysis, or to rational justification. As to this tendency to believe that there is a spiritual order in the universe, and to feel that he personally has a stake in the world process, man cannot say much more than

> We have but faith; we cannot know,
> For knowledge is of things we see;
> And yet we trust it comes from thee,
> A beam in darkness; let it grow.

76

To many the presentation of beliefs as adaptive mechanisms is unpalatable; beliefs from this point of view would be individual, opportunistic, utilitarian, shifting, relative. Many want something more solid on which to build their intellectual and moral universe, something which they can feel is not merely relatively useful but absolutely right. The discussion of the meaning of absolute rightness would lead us into a rare atmosphere of metaphysical discussion, in which the biologist finds respiration difficult. The quest for an absolute guaranty of rightness suggests the haunting desire for security and protection, which harks back to the early experience of the child in the protective atmosphere of the home. All, however, are not preoccupied to the same degree with this desire for security; some are content with the feeling of conviction associated with those beliefs which enable them best to work out the purposes with which they have identified themselves. Such an attitude involves a certain independence and spirit of adventure, a willingness to do the best one can with one's personal experience, a complete acceptance of personal responsibility.

This attitude may shock the timid who require the moral support of the absolute, it may seem crude to those skilled in the logical and metaphysical distillation of truth; from the point of view of the health of the individual and of the social group, there is much to commend it.

It is obvious that the partial analysis given above of the underlying conditions of belief has not led to a very definite goal; but the journey may not have been without gain. Setting out to reach, if possible, something final, static, absolute in the realm of belief, one finds that beliefs are the tools of life, rather than rare intellectual products to be carefully cherished for themselves. What beliefs may thus seem to lose in prestige they gain in their value for life, and their significance is seen in the light of the strivings of the individual. The right mode of life and right beliefs are problems too intimately interwoven to be thought of apart, and he who searches for right beliefs is also searching for the right way of life; in both directions the individual cannot transcend the limits of his endowment or get beyond what is relative.

While it is not possible for anyone to transcend the limits of his endowment or attain the absolute, it may be possible for him to eliminate, or make the necessary correction for, certain distorting factors in the personal equation, such as constitutional traits, disturbing experiences in the past, borrowed attitudes and emotional values, strong underlying trends, moral laziness and cowardice. A systematic review of one's personality with the aim of modifying an undue subjectivity is no mere intellectual diversion, it is a dynamic process involving a new orientation toward experience, which makes the resources of the individual more fully available for the tasks of life, and the same fuller utilization of resources may be the reward of that state or nation which does not hesitate to review its cherished social beliefs and institutions.